Nibbles
of
Encouragement

Nibbles
of
Encouragement

**Small Bites of Encouragement, Inspiration, and
Reinforcement to Help You on
Your Weight Loss Journey**

By

George A. Diamond

A & C Publishing
AC-Publishing.com

Published 2013 by A & C Publishing
© Copyright 2013 George A. Diamond
AC-Publishing.com

ISBN-13: 978-0-615-79583-6

Dedication

I dedicate this book to all those who have a strong desire to lose weight and who are planning their Weight Loss Journey.

It is the author's experience that those who read this book have a strong desire to lose weight.

Acknowledgments

Writing a book involves a lot of time and work. Therefore, I would like to thank the following people for their role in helping to make this book a reality.

First of all, I want to thank my wife Jane, and children Anthony and Christopher for their support and patience while writing this book.

I want to thank my parents, my father the late George K. Diamond and my mother Mary Diamond, for their guidance, encouragement and the solid foundation for life which they gave me as I was growing up.

Introduction

Losing weight is about developing a thin person mind-set. It is about making the choices that a thin person would make. It is about getting rid of our excuses, overcoming weight-loss obstacles, and developing lifelong motivation.

This can be rewarding, but it can also be challenging and frustrating at times. However, the right words at the right time can keep us on the right track. The right words can help us stay focused. The right words can also keep us committed to our weight-loss goal.

There will be times that we will feel discouraged. We will find that we need a little inspiration and encouragement to keep us going. It can be as simple as an inspirational quote to get us back on track.

It is the author's hope that *Nibbles of Encouragement* will inspire us to make the right choices daily. It is the extra edge we need, to have success at losing weight. *Nibbles of Encouragement* contains powerful words that the author has used to help countless people reach their weight-loss goals.

It is suggested that this book be read many times as we go through the weight-loss process. We should memorize the quotes that inspire us or even write them and cycle them through our mind. Repeat these nibbles to ourselves as often as situations arise. Weight-loss success is only a few pages away.

WE CAN DO IT!!!

2

Nibbles of Encouragement

(1)
What is our health and ultimately our life worth?

~~~~~~~~~~

(2)
First, we need to be aware, of how we spend our time, and then make time for what's truly important. It should be our health.

~~~~~~~~~~

(3)
Losing weight is about moving in a positive direction. We do this by making one right decision after another.

~~~~~~~~~~

(4)
I found that losing weight was difficult when I had an, "I can't lose weight" attitude. If I wanted to lose weight, I knew that I needed to lose that attitude. Will you? These nibbles may help you as long as you keep an open mind.

3

(5)

Anyone can lose weight once they remove any doubt they have about their ability to become thinner. This is because once the doubt is gone; they will be able to make the smart choices so that they can lose the weight they desire.

~~~~~~~~~~

(6)

I found for myself that it was important to make it a point to do a few things each day that moved me towards weight loss and fitness that I may not have wanted to do. How about you?

~~~~~~~~~~

(7)

If we want to lose weight, it is important to fight our initial thoughts and feelings about weight loss.

~~~~~~~~~~

(8)

Losing weight is usually difficult at the beginning, but it will eventually become easier.

(9)

What attitude should we have if we want to lose weight? We should be unhappy with our weight yet excited that we can do something about it.

~~~~~~~~~~

(10)

It is important to know the REALITY of our weight problem. Are we happy with it? If not, we need to use that dissatisfaction to move us in a positive direction. Extreme dissatisfaction can be a powerful motivator that can be used as our "Reason Why."

~~~~~~~~~~

(11)

It is always a great idea to make an investment in our health. The longer we wait, the longer we will be overweight and possibly unhealthy.

~~~~~~~~~~

(12)

We need to understand that we cannot eat like we used to, and expect to not gain weight. Therefore, we must know, think, and believe that we cannot continue the old habits!

(13)

Set big weight loss and fitness goals, and then break them down into smaller manageable goals.

~~~~~~~~~

(14)

Be careful. Most people don't decide to stop losing weight. They just slowly revert back to their old bad habits.

~~~~~~~~~

(15)

People fail at losing weight because they have stopped doing what they have committed to themselves that they would do.

~~~~~~~~~

(16)

What do we need to do today to lose weight and get fit, but have been putting off? Let's do it today. We will be glad we did.

(17)

Let's ask ourselves, "What were my setbacks in losing weight and getting fit? What did I learn from those setbacks? How can I avoid them in the future?"

~~~~~~~~~~

(18)

I was not able to lose weight until I got rid of the wrong thinking I had towards food, weight loss, and fitness. Will you be able to get rid of your wrong thinking?

~~~~~~~~~~

(19)

We should always focus on the result, and how losing weight will affect our lives. This is what I like to call our "REASON WHY."

~~~~~~~~~~

(20)

Do not procrastinate. Let's get started, and always keep our weight loss and fitness moving forward in a positive direction.

(21)

Expect obstacles and challenges during the weight-loss process. They are part of the process. However, consistency and persistence will win every time.

~~~~~~~~~~~

(22)

It takes some effort to lose weight. However, it can easily be gained back if we lose our focus.

~~~~~~~~~~~

(23)

If we don't like our weight, we can do something about it! I did. I lost 50 pounds in four months and have kept it off for seven years, how about you?

~~~~~~~~~~~

(24)

The only thing keeping anyone from losing weight is the power of their desire to do it.

(25)

We didn't gain the weight overnight. Why should we expect to lose it overnight? It will take patience and effort to lose the weight we want.

~~~~~~~~~~

(26)

I did not play around with losing weight. I figured if I did not take it seriously I won't get anywhere. Taking weight loss seriously will help us reach our goal.

~~~~~~~~~~

(27)

Small positive changes in our habits can make a positive impact on our weight.

~~~~~~~~~~

(28)

Weight loss is a life long journey and an education. It is not the destination. We learn what to do and what not to do along the way.

(29)

What are we going to do today to move towards our weight-loss goal?

~~~~~~~~~~

(30)

I have never had anyone tell me that they regretted losing weight.
However, I have had people tell me they regretted not losing it.

~~~~~~~~~~

(31)

We can choose a thin future over an overweight past. It is a choice. It is
our choice. Make the right choice.

~~~~~~~~~~

(32)

We need to be positive that we can lose the weight we desire. A
positive attitude is a key to weight loss.

(33)

We can trade the short-term gratification that food gives us for a long term healthier future. Let's make the trade.

~~~~~~~~~~~

(34)

Forget about the weight-loss problems of the past. What matters is what we are going to do about it now and in the future.

~~~~~~~~~~~

(35)

Positive weight-loss actions result in weight-loss success.

~~~~~~~~~~~

(36)

Weight-loss success is related to our drive to become thinner and healthier.

(37)

If we take consistent action, and stay focused, we will lose the weight we desire.

~~~~~~~~~~

(38)

We need to take responsibility for our weight-loss results.

~~~~~~~~~~

(39)

People that are successful at losing weight, make the right choices.

~~~~~~~~~~

(40)

People that lose weight don't make excuses.

(41)

If what we are doing to lose weight is not working, we need to do something different.

~~~~~~~~~

(42)

We will not lose weight without overcoming obstacles. It is part of the weight-loss process.

~~~~~~~~~

(43)

Weight-loss success is an accumulation of small positive and consistent actions.

~~~~~~~~~

(44)

We can't lose weight and keep it off, unless we enjoy the process.

(45)

We need to identify the reasons for our past weight-loss failures and develop new plans, so they don't happen in the future.

~~~~~~~~~~~

(46)

Losing weight is about doing things that most overweight people won't do.

~~~~~~~~~~~

(47)

Let's lose weight and be an inspiration to everyone around us (our partner, our children, our grandchildren, our friends).

~~~~~~~~~~~

(48)

There are no shortcuts to losing weight, let's not spend our valuable time looking for them.

(49)

Weight loss will only happen if we make it happen.

~~~~~~~~~~

(50)

Weight loss happens for those who are the most determined.

~~~~~~~~~~

(51)

Our ability to lose weight is based on our readiness to do it.

~~~~~~~~~~

(52)

Part of losing weight is keeping focused on our weight-loss goal.

(53)

Fitness takes time. However, the investment of time to exercise is an investment in our health and our future.

~~~~~~~~~~

(54)

If I wanted to lose weight, I knew I would have to be willing to do the small things it took to lose weight. Are you willing to do the small things it takes to lose weight? It can be going for a walk after dinner. It can be packing a lighter and healthier lunch. It can be not going up for seconds at mealtime. These are a few of the little things that can really make the difference.

~~~~~~~~~~

(55)

Losing weight is not one method fits all. Therefore, we need to ask ourselves, "How can I lose weight?" The answer may be what we need.

~~~~~~~~~~

(56)

Those who are successful at losing weight, look for opportunities to exercise. Unsuccessful people find excuses to avoid it.

(57)

If we want to be successful at losing weight, we must start.

~~~~~~~~~~

(58)

If we want to lose weight, we must have the right mindset towards it.

~~~~~~~~~~

(59)

Laziness can be an obstacle to losing weight. Don't let it be.

~~~~~~~~~~

(60)

To lose weight, we need to set a weight-loss goal. If we don't have a goal, we won't lose weight. However, if we have a big weight-loss goal, we can lose a lot of weight. Therefore, let's set a big weight-loss goal and let's get started.

(61)

Total focus on our weight-loss goal means total commitment. When we have total focus and total commitment, we will lose weight.

~~~~~~~~~~

(62)

Daily positive steps towards losing weight are essential for weight-loss success.

~~~~~~~~~~

(63)

Planning for retirement does not just mean planning our finances. It also means planning for the health we would like to enjoy with those finances.

~~~~~~~~~~

(64)

There are many keys to losing weight. Diligence towards our weight-loss goal is one of them.

(65)

We need to look at our current weight. Look at our future with that weight. If we don't like what we see, change it before it is too late.

~~~~~~~~~~

(66)

There is only one person who can stop us from losing weight. That person is ourselves.

~~~~~~~~~~

(67)

Positive daily actions are a key to positive weight-loss results.

~~~~~~~~~~

(68)

All the weight-loss tips and secrets in the world won't work until we actually internalize them and do them.

(69)

The road to weight-loss success is always filled with obstacles waiting to send us back to our old bad habits.

~~~~~~~~~~

(70)

A secret to weight-loss success is to work hard at losing weight and don't ever quit.

~~~~~~~~~~

(71)

Making trade-offs is a key to having weight-loss success. We can trade being thinner and having knees that don't hurt by avoiding French fries. We can trade not getting diabetes by replacing soda with water. There are many tradeoffs we can make everyday, once we think about the possibilities.

~~~~~~~~~~

(72)

People that fail at losing weight usually lack the motivation to do it.

(73)

A healthy future belongs to those who work towards it.

~~~~~~~~~~

(74)

A person's level of determination to lose weight, will determine their success or failure.

~~~~~~~~~~

(75)

Fear of the weight-loss process can keep us overweight.

~~~~~~~~~~

(76)

I realized a long time ago that I was the only one who could keep me from starting the weight-loss process. I also realized that I was the only one who could cause me to fail or succeed at losing weight. It was all up to me.

(77)

I found that I could change a weight-loss failure into a success just by coming at it from a different angle. You can too.

~~~~~~~~~~

(78)

We will never be able to lose weight until we are ready to go after it.

~~~~~~~~~~

(79)

Weight loss will not come to those who procrastinate but to those who work at it.

~~~~~~~~~~

(80)

When we keep working at losing weight, and don't stop, we will not fail.

(81)

Weight loss usually doesn't happen on its own. We have to make it happen.

~~~~~~~~~~

(82)

On the weight-loss journey, we will have many disappointments. The question is, "What are we going to do about them? Are we going to quit or are we going to keep moving forward?" It is all up to us.

~~~~~~~~~~

(83)

Weight-loss success is based on the things we do. Positive actions will give us positive results. Negative actions will give us negative results.

~~~~~~~~~~

(84)

The concept of weight-loss success is simple. We need to eat less and get more exercise if we want to lose weight. What are we waiting for? Let's get going.

(85)

Some people dream of being thinner while others just go do it. Let's stop dreaming about being thinner and do it. Let's turn our dream into a reality.

~~~~~~~~~~

(86)

Losing weight and sitting on the sofa don't go together.

~~~~~~~~~~

(87)

Weight loss doesn't come to us. We must chase after it.

~~~~~~~~~~

(88)

Don't just talk about losing weight, just do it.

(89)

The best way to lose weight is to enjoy losing weight and have fun with it. This will help keep the motivation strong.

~~~~~~~~~~

(90)

Weight loss can be uneasy for us before it becomes easy.

~~~~~~~~~~

(91)

The hard part of losing weight is starting. Let's get started and watch the weight come off.

~~~~~~~~~~

(92)

To be successful at losing weight, we must be ready to win.

(93)

We need to do things daily that concern, our weight and our fitness, if we want weight-loss success.

~~~~~~~~~~

(94)

We can do what it takes to lose weight. The question is "WILL WE?"

~~~~~~~~~~

(95)

The desire alone to lose weight will not make it happen. We also need to do something about it.

~~~~~~~~~~

(96)

The best time to start losing weight is now. Don't wait. Start now.

(97)

One of the things that we need to do is to look in the mirror and ask ourselves this question, "Have I gained just a couple of pounds or do I have a weight problem?" We usually won't notice a couple of extra pounds. Additionally, admitting we have a weight problem will put more importance on losing it.

~~~~~~~~~~

(98)

Don't concentrate on the weight problem; concentrate on what can be done to solve the weight problem.

~~~~~~~~~~

(99)

When I was overweight, I found that going through the day, overweight and out of shape, was like towing my boat everywhere I went. It wasn't easy. If you are overweight, it is probably not easy for you either. Therefore, let's do something about it.

~~~~~~~~~~

(100)

Let's look at the successes we've had in losing weight. This can help us make better choices now and in the future.

(101)
Losing weight is possible if we truly hope and believe it is.

~~~~~~~~~~

(102)
Let's prepare our health for the future. It starts with being at a healthy weight.

~~~~~~~~~~

(103)
Let's start taking control of our present and future health by taking control of our weight.

~~~~~~~~~~

(104)
Not deciding to lose weight and get fit is a decision. Therefore, let's make the right decision and let's get started.

(105)

It is possible to lose weight if we choose. We just have to make the choice.

~~~~~~~~~~

(106)

Don't try to lose weight, just do it.

~~~~~~~~~~

(107)

Our present and future daily choices, determine our future weight and health.

~~~~~~~~~~

(108)

Let's lead our families, let's lose weight, and let's set the example that our children and grandchildren can follow.

(109)

We need to keep our focus on where we want our weight to be, and not on the things it takes to get there. In other words, we need to focus on the goal not the process.

~~~~~~~~~~

(110)

Today is the first day of our future weight and future health. What would we like our future health to be like? The answer can help motivate us.

~~~~~~~~~~

(111)

It is a great idea to monitor our weight daily so that we can see the results of our daily choices.

~~~~~~~~~~

(112)

Exercise should not be looked at as pain, work, or sweat. It should be looked at as fun and play. If we have fun with it, we will do it for life.

(113)

Weight-loss success is attained by those who commit to working at it until they succeed.

~~~~~~~~~~

(114)

If we want to lose weight, we will need to make weight loss our number-one priority.

~~~~~~~~~~

(115)

We should not treat losing weight like a hobby. We should treat losing weight like a daily emergency.

~~~~~~

(116)

We need to be mindful of our daily choices because those decisions will determine our future health.

(117)

Most people plan and prepare when they go on vacation. How about planning and preparing so that we can have a long and healthy future?

~~~~~~~~~

(118)

Weight-loss failure only occurs when we decide to stop.

~~~~~~~~~

(119)

We can lose weight if we have the enthusiasm to do it.

~~~~~~~~~

(120)

A wish or desire to lose weight does not make us thinner. A decision to lose weight followed by positive action is the key.

(121)

We should ignore anyone who tells us that we can't lose weight. They are just talking about themselves. Remember misery likes company.

~~~~~~~~~~

(122)

I found that since I made exercise fun, I look forward to it. I hope you will also!

~~~~~~~~~~

(123)

A great way to lose weight is to stay focused on the "Reason Why" we want to lose it.

~~~~~~~~~~

(124)

We always need to take responsibility for our daily choices.

(125)
We always need to let go of our past weight-loss failures. They can keep us overweight.

~~~~~~~~~~

(126)
If we have time to whine about our weight, we can make the time to lose it.

~~~~~~~~~~

(127)
If we don't believe that we can lose weight, we will never lose it.

~~~~~~~~~~

(128)
Let's not focus on what has happened to our past weight-loss attempts. Focus only on our thin and fit future, along with what we need to do to get there.

(129)

Hope is powerful. Have strong hope that we can lose weight, and we can. If we are hopeless, we won't.

~~~~~~~~~~

(130)

Do you have a dream of being thinner and fitter like I did? It can be done. We need to know that we can do it. We need to work at it daily. Lastly, it is important to keep working towards that dream and never stop until you succeed.

~~~~~~~~~~

(131)

All of us who have lost weight have made mistakes during the weight-loss process. Don't worry if you make a weight-loss mistake. It will happen. It is important to learn from those mistakes so that we don't repeat them.

~~~~~~~~~~

(132)

There was one moment when I looked into the mirror and wondered, "What happened? How did I let myself get this way?" I then decided that I could do something about it. How about you? Have you found your moment?

(133)

People fail at losing weight because they are concentrating on the weight-loss process instead of the results.

~~~~~~~~~~

(134)

One of the best ways to fight old age is by being thin and fit. It can make us look and feel younger.

~~~~~~~~~~

(135)

When is the perfect time to start losing weight? THE TIME IS NOW. The longer we wait, the closer we will be to having irreversible health issues.

~~~~~~~~~~

(136)

The question is not, "If we think we are overweight or how we became overweight?" The question is, "Are we going to do anything about it?"

(137)

Everyday we need to say to ourselves, "I know I can lose weight. I know I can lose weight. I know I can lose weight …"

~~~~~~~~~

(138)

When we get upset and are ready to stop losing weight, remember that we are closer to our weight-loss goal than we think.

~~~~~~~~~

(139)

People spend their time doing what they feel is important. If our health is important, we will make the time to lose weight and get fit.

~~~~~~~~~

(140)

It is important for us not to give ourselves any trouble over losing weight and getting fit.

(141)

We can be in control of losing weight and changing our future health, or we can lose our health and let it control us. It is our choice.

~~~~~~~~~~~

(142)

The people who are successful at losing weight look forward to a thinner future.

~~~~~~~~~~~

(143)

It is important for us to start every day with a plan that will move us towards our weight loss and fitness goals.

~~~~~~~~~~~

(144)

It is important not to accept being overweight. Let's start by controlling our future health, our weight, and our fitness.

(145)

If we don't make our health number one, we won't be around for
anything else.

~~~~~~~~~

(146)

When I started to lose weight, I asked myself, "I can lose weight if I do
what?" The answer was enlightening. Your answer can be
enlightening also.

~~~~~~~~~

(147)

Do we focus our attention on the past, the present, or the future?
It is important to focus our attention on the future, not the past, nor the
present. We must see a thin future for ourselves and focus our attention
and effort on getting there.

~~~~~~~~~

(148)

Before we can lose the weight we want, we need to know the weight
we want to be. That is why it is first important to set a goal.

(149)

If we are going to be stubborn about something let's be stubborn about losing weight.

~~~~~~~~~

(150)

Don't ever quit losing weight, we can do it!

~~~~~~~~~

(151)

We will have obstacles in our way during the weight-loss process. Our character will determine our response. Will we quit or will it drive us to win at losing weight?

~~~~~~~~~

(152)

We should not wait for a heart attack or a stroke before we take our health seriously.

(153)

Losing weight goes to those who are the most persistent.

~~~~~~~~~~

(154)

We usually get what we ask for. Therefore, we should not ask for poor health by abusing our bodies.

~~~~~~~~~~

(155)

If we believe in ourselves and start losing weight and getting fit, the thinner us will come out.

~~~~~~~~~~

(156)

Let's not underestimate the power of our commitments to ourselves. Therefore, let's make the decision to lose weight and then commit to that decision.

41

(157)

I always hear people say that they are trying to lose weight. However, their actions tell a different story. It is better to lose weight than just to talk about it.

~~~~~~~~~~

(158)

It takes courage to do the things we may not want to do, to lose weight.

~~~~~~~~~~

(159)

There will be things that will try to stop us during the weight-loss process. It is how we deal with them that will determine our success or failure.

~~~~~~~~~~

(160)

Eating junk food is not the problem. Eating more than a taste is. It takes strength and commitment not to eat more than a taste.

(161)

A person cannot lose weight without overcoming obstacles and challenges.

~~~~~~~~~~

(162)

Be willing to pay the price to get and stay healthy. It is a small price to pay.

~~~~~~~~~~

(163)

Overeating is usually an emotional release. Try exercising instead. It works!

~~~~~~~~~~

(164)

All of us have the ability to lose weight, now all we need is the motivation and attitude, and we will succeed.

(165)

People need to realize that a half-hour walk does not cancel overeating.

~~~~~~~~~~~~

(166)

We must know that we can make daily progress towards losing weight, before we can lose weight and get fit.

~~~~~~~~~~~~

(167)

The weight-loss process can be tough until it becomes a habit.

~~~~~~~~~~~~

(168)

One of the first steps in the weight-loss process is to make the decision to lose weight for the last time.

(169)

Before we can lose weight, we need to ask ourselves, "What are my priorities and how do I spend my time?" If we think about it, more priority should be placed on our weight, health, and fitness.

~~~~~~~~~~

(170)

Exercise is a great replacement for emotional eating.

~~~~~~~~~~

(171)

Let's spend some of our valuable time on our valuable health, and let's lose weight and get fit.

~~~~~~~~~~

(172)

Here are a few easy ways we can make time in our day to exercise:
1. Wake up earlier and exercise.
2. Go to bed later and use that extra time to exercise.
3. Walk or exercise during lunch.
4. Turn our TV time into exercise time.

(173)

We can make the quick gratification decisions and have a painful future, or we can lose weight, and have an easier and less painful future. I opt for the second, because losing weight is a lot less painful than health issues. How about you?

~~~~~~~~~~

(174)

We need to keep going after weight loss until we decide to win.

~~~~~~~~~~

(175)

We will never have success at losing weight, if we never go for it.

~~~~~~~~~~

(176)

If we don't start losing weight, we will never become thinner.

(177)

Weight-loss success and positive weight-loss action are related. So let's get started.

~~~~~~~~~~

(178)

Weight loss happens when what we believe, what we think, what we say, and what we do, are aligned.

~~~~~~~~~~

(179)

Positive weight-loss actions from us, creates positive weight-loss actions by those around us.

~~~~~~~~~~

(180)

Complete this sentence: "I can lose weight with…"

(181)

Our opportunity to lose weight is ringing. Are we going to answer or let it go into voicemail?

~~~~~~~~~~

(182)

If we want to lose weight, we will need to do what we have not been willing to do in the past.

~~~~~~~~~~

(183)

We should not worry about our weight-loss problem. It is a problem that we can do something about. Let's get started.

~~~~~~~~~~

(184)

We need to admit that we have a weight problem and then start to deal with it. There is nothing positive that comes from ignoring or denying the problem.

(185)

Don't ever think that weight loss is impossible, it is possible and achievable.

~~~~~~~~~

(186)

Asking ourselves a question can sometimes give us some insight into why we are not losing weight. Let's ask ourselves, "I can lose weight after I..?

~~~~~~~~~

(187)

Just because we are overweight that does not mean that we can't lose it.

~~~~~~~~~

(188)

Make the decision to lose weight then commit to that decision. That's the power of losing weight.

(189)

It is a great idea to ask ourselves, "Do we hate being overweight?" If the answer is "YES," then let's do something about it.

~~~~~~~~~~~

(190)

The few minutes of satisfaction we get out of eating that junk food, causes us to suffer from that point on (i.e. sore knees, diabetes, high blood pressure, etc.). Is it worth it? It wasn't for me.

~~~~~~~~~~~

(191)

No one can motivate us to lose weight. We must motivate ourselves. Motivation comes from within.

~~~~~~~~~~~

(192)

The greater number of things that we do towards our weight-loss goal, the bigger results we will have.

(193)

Weight-loss success is attained by those who keep working at it.

~~~~~~~~~

(194)

We should be vain about our looks and use that vanity to our advantage as we lose weight.

~~~~~~~~~

(195)

An obstacle to losing weight is our ability to change the doubt in our mind that *we can do it*.

~~~~~~~~~

(196)

As we lose weight, we need to think about all the things we will be able to do when we are thinner. What are the things you want to do?

(197)

We should not be impatient when it comes to losing weight. We don't need the frustration. Remember, the weight did not go on overnight.

~~~~~~~~~

(198)

If we want weight-loss success, we need to refuse to stop trying.

~~~~~~~~~

(199)

Do not put off losing weight because it looks hard.

~~~~~~~~~

(200)

If we have the right attitude, there is nothing that will keep us from losing weight.

(201)

If we want to lose weight, we must be self-motivated to succeed. This means that we will refuse to fail.

~~~~~~~~~~~

(202)

There will be many road blocks during the weight-loss process. They are part of the process. How we handle our weight-loss road blocks will determine our failure or success.

~~~~~~~~~~~

(203)

Most people don't lose weight the first time. The key is to keep at it until we succeed.

~~~~~~~~~~~

(204)

People who fail at losing weight concentrate on the obstacles that get in their way. People who succeed at losing weight concentrate on finding solutions around those obstacles.

(205)

We won't lose weight if we think we can't.

~~~~~~~~~~

(206)

The decision to lose weight can cause some anxiety, but it is worth it.

~~~~~~~~~~

(207)

Trade-offs are part of the weight-loss process. We can't lose weight without them.

~~~~~~~~~~

(208)

Weight-loss success depends on what we think about food, exercise, and the weight-loss process.

(209)

We will not be able to lose weight on what we are going to do in the future. "I am going to lose weight after...." This will do nothing to help us lose weight now.

~~~~~~~~~~

(210)

If we want to lose weight, we will need to find a way to enjoy it.

~~~~~~~~~~

(211)

Learning from our weight-loss setbacks is an essential part of losing weight.

~~~~~~~~~~

(212)

Daily progress needs to be part of our weight-loss plan if we want to lose weight.

(213)

Weight-loss failures can either force us to quit or drive us to succeed. Which one will it be for you?

~~~~~~~~~~

(214)

A strong desire to lose weight is a great place to start.

~~~~~~~~~~

(215)

Losing weight should not be thought of as scary. It should be something that we look forward to. Think about what it would be like to be thinner and get excited to get started.

~~~~~~~~~~

(216)

Make a game out of losing weight. Let's challenge ourselves and have fun with it.

(217)

Our car would not run well putting water in the gas tank. Our bodies will not run well when we fuel it with junk food. The difference between our car and our body is that if we ruin our car, we can always buy another one. We can't buy a new body.

~~~~~~~~~

(218)

Most people feel fear when they are making the decision to lose weight. We will need to deal with this fear, or we will not succeed at losing weight.

~~~~~~~~~

(219)

When I was in the weight-loss process, I tried a lot of different things. Some things worked. Some things didn't work. However, what I learned in the process was extremely valuable.

~~~~~~~~~

(220)

If we keep failing at losing weight, we need to look at what we are doing. If we have been doing the same thing over and over with no results, then the answer is simple. We need to try something different. A different approach can give us different results.

(221)

We will never get thinner until we are ready to do something about our overeating and lack of exercise.

~~~~~~~~~~

(222)

Don't like to sweat? There are many exercises that we can do that don't require sweating. Walking is one of them. Now what's our excuse?

~~~~~~~~~~

(223)

The heavier we are, the less mobile we will be in the future. Choose a healthier, thinner, and more mobile future today. Let's start by losing weight.

~~~~~~~~~~

(224)

If we are overweight and don't like how we feel, losing weight may be the key.

(225)

Losing weight is a great way to control our health. The alternative is that our health will control us.

~~~~~~~~~~

(226)

Don't blame our genetics. It's our daily choices not our genetics that determines our weight.

~~~~~~~~~~

(227)

The decision to losing weight is the most important decision we will ever make. Make it once and get it done.

~~~~~~~~~~

(228)

Admitting we have a weight problem is the beginning of the weight-loss process.

(229)

The education we get during the weight-loss process will keep us thin after we lose the weight. If we don't learn anything during the process, we will gain the weight back.

~~~~~~~~~

(230)

Never pass by an opportunity to burn more calories.

~~~~~~~~~

(231)

The best way to lose weight is to set a goal.

~~~~~~~~~

(232)

Learning why we eat and don't exercise can help give us the power to lose weight.

(233)

We will need to change our negative thoughts towards weight loss to positive ones if we want to lose weight.

~~~~~~~~~~

(234)

Our eating and exercise habits will decide our future.

~~~~~~~~~~

(235)

Would it be easier getting dressed in the morning if we were thinner? If the answer is "YES," then let's do something about it.

~~~~~~~~~~

(236)

Do we think losing weight is hard? It will continue to be hard until we change that attitude. Losing weight is as hard or easy as we make it.

(237)

The weight-loss process can be painful or exciting; it's how we look at it.

~~~~~~~~~

(238)

Let's overcome our weight-loss stumbling blocks and succeed.

~~~~~~~~~

(239)

Let's picture ourselves with a thinner future, and let's do what it takes to get to that future. Think of all the things that we would be able to do easier than we can do today.

~~~~~~~~~

(240)

If we can put enough pressure on ourselves, we will lose weight.

(241)

Making the changes in our lives that we need to make to lose weight and keeping it off can be scary. However, this fear is normal but needs to be replaced with anticipation and excitement, if we want to succeed.

~~~~~~~~~~

(242)

Think of losing weight as going on a vacation. Look forward to it, plan for it, and don't concentrate on all the stuff we need to do to lose weight. Just concentrate on the results.

~~~~~~~~~~

(243)

There is always some discouragement from time to time during the weight-loss process. Realize that it is normal, keep moving forward, and succeed.

~~~~~~~~~~

(244)

Self-pity is an enemy of weight loss. It will keep us overweight and unhappy, if we let it.

(245)

We all have the ability to get to the weight that we will be happy to live with the rest of our life.

~~~~~~~~~~

(246)

The process of losing weight will also show us a lot about ourselves. Make it a positive experience.

~~~~~~~~~~

(247)

What are we going to do today towards losing weight and transforming our lives?

~~~~~~~~~~

(248)

After I lost 30 of the 50 pounds, overweight people told me I lost too much weight. Remember that misery likes company. We should not ask other people for permission because we may not always get it. Our doctor is the only person we should listen to about how much weight we should lose.

(249)

We will not be able to get thinner by staying in our comfort zone and clinging to our excuses. People always tell me:
"I'm too busy to exercise."
"I don't like to sweat."
"Exercise is too much work."
It is time to get out of our comfort zone, lose those excuses, start exercising, and lose weight.

~~~~~~~~~~

(250)

Life can be taken from us at any time. Let's do what we can to take care of ourselves so that we can live a long and healthy life.

~~~~~~~~~~

(251)

Lose weight and surprise all the people that say that we can't do it.

~~~~~~~~~~

(252)

Those who are overweight will try to discourage our weight-loss plans. Don't let them.

(253)

Put a quick weight-loss plan together, get started, and let's modify it as we go.

~~~~~~~~~

(254)

If we don't have a plan for our health, we will be part of someone else's financial plan (i.e. fast-food restaurants, junk food companies, etc.). They benefit financially from our poor habits.

~~~~~~~~~

(255)

We need to say to ourselves: "I let myself get this way. I will do what needs to be done to get the weight off."

~~~~~~~~~

(256)

Do not settle for staying overweight. Staying content is a great way to go nowhere fast.

(257)

The day we stop making excuses is the day we start to lose weight.

~~~~~~~~~~

(258)

Place our daily weight, exercise, and other healthy activities on our calendar. Calendaring any activity gives it priority.

~~~~~~~~~~

(259)

The key to getting fit is giving our cardiovascular system a good workout. We can play a sport, go for a power walk, or go to the gym. It will help our cardiovascular system, boost our metabolism, and help reduce our stress.

~~~~~~~~~~

(260)

Let's add enjoyment to our weight loss and our weight loss experience will be an enjoyable and positive one.

(261)

Let's not let justifications and distractions keep our weight where it is. This will cause us to trade our future health for the excuse of the day.

~~~~~~~~~~

(262)

The decision to lose weight is the biggest decision we can make for our health and our future.

~~~~~~~~~~

(263)

A negative attitude will not allow us to lose weight, but a positive attitude can. So let's have a positive attitude about losing weight and let's get started.

~~~~~~~~~~

(264)

Losing weight is not about what you can't have. It is about what you will be able to have once you lose it (better health, better mobility, etc...).

(265)

We can lose weight or we can make excuses why we can't. The first is more rewarding.

~~~~~~~~~~

(266)

Don't focus on being overweight. Focus on what we need to do to get it off.

~~~~~~~~~~

(267)

Let's gain control of our eating habits, and our exercising habits so that we can gain control of our lives.

~~~~~~~~~~

(268)

We need to prepare mentally for the task of losing weight, and we need to have a plan, before we can succeed at it.

(269)

Don't be scared of how slowly you may lose weight; be scared of not losing any weight or not starting the process at all.

~~~~~~~~~

(270)

We should not get mad when we make a mistake during the weight-loss process. We should learn from it and don't make it a second time.

~~~~~~~~~

(271)

When I was in the weight-loss process, I was amazed at all the advice I got from overweight people. What advice would we give someone about losing weight if we had the chance? Let's listen to our own advice and start losing weight today.

~~~~~~~~~

(272)

Weight-loss success is like walking. We take one step at a time, and eventually we end up where we want to be.

(273)

We should not avoid losing weight today because we may not be able to avoid the health problems it will give us in the future.

~~~~~~~~~~

(274)

The weight-loss process is about the journey not the destination. It is about having one small success after another until we succeed.

~~~~~~~~~~

(275)

Our bad/unhealthy eating habits have to disappear if we want to manage our weight, and only we can overcome them.

~~~~~~~~~~

(276)

Changing how we eat can be hard. However, it is doable and well worth it.

(277)

When I was in the weight-loss process I would constantly ask myself, "Is what I am about to eat taking me towards or away from my weight-loss goal?"

~~~~~~~~~~

(278)

We don't lose weight with luck. It takes a plan and lots of right choices.

~~~~~~~~~~

(279)

Let's not be remembered as someone who lacked self-control.

~~~~~~~~~~

(280)

If we overeat now we will pay for it later.

(281)

A person who loses weight does things that overweight people refuse to do.

~~~~~~~~~~

(282)

Let's not ignore the fact that if we don't lose weight, our odds of having health problems increase. Ignoring this fact will not change the future.

~~~~~~~~~~

(283)

We will get off the weight-loss track when we say "YES" to the wrong things.

~~~~~~~~~~

(284)

We can lose weight if we trade instant gratification for a thinner and healthier future.

(285)

If we make weight loss important, it will keep us motivated.

~~~~~~~~~

(286)

We can have good intensions to lose weight, but without doing something about it, our weight-loss results won't change.

~~~~~~~~~

(287)

Are we moving in the direction of a healthier future? If not, it's time to change course.

~~~~~~~~~

(288)

Our actions, not our words, will show how serious we are about losing weight.

(289)

If we start making slight changes in both our food and exercise routines, we will see the weight come off.

~~~~~~~~~~

(290)

We can lose weight and move into a healthier future, or stay overweight and move into a future of health issues. It's our choice.

~~~~~~~~~~

(291)

There are a lot of things that we cannot control. However, we should not refuse to do something that we have control over, and that is to lose weight and get more fit.

~~~~~~~~~~

(292)

The first step in losing weight is that we must admit to ourselves that we need to lose weight. We then need to decide to do something about it.

75

(293)

Eighty-five percent of the challenge to losing weight is getting and keeping our motivation. The other fifteen percent is making it happen.

~~~~~~~~~

(294)

Weight-loss success is the result of exercising regularly and burning more calories than we take in.

~~~~~~~~~

(295)

We should not ignore the ability we have to lose weight and get fit.

~~~~~~~~~

(296)

If we truly know and believe that we can lose weight. I truly believe that we can do it.

(297)

If we can't lose weight fast, we need to take it in small and consistent steps, and we will succeed.

~~~~~~~~~~

(298)

Most weight-loss obstacles are ones that we create and most of them live only in our head.

~~~~~~~~~~

(299)

Having a "Reason Why" for losing weight is the ultimate motivator.

~~~~~~~~~~

(300)

Do we deserve to lose weight? We will be tested along the way. We will have obstacles put in front of us. We will make weight-loss mistakes. There will be times we will have little or no results. Pass these tests and we will lose weight.

(301)

The food and exercise decisions we've made, until now, got us to where our weight is today. Our food and decisions from this day forwards, will determine our weight in the future.

~~~~~~~~~~

(302)

Self gratification will not allow us to get thinner because it trades the now for the future. Losing weight is about trading the future for the now.

~~~~~~~~~~

(303)

Thinking thin thoughts will allow us to do things a thin person would do so that we can lose weight.

~~~~~~~~~~

(304)

The best thing that we can do if we make mistakes during the weight-loss process is to forgive ourselves and keep going forward.

(305)

Losing weight is all about having the right mind-set.

~~~~~~~~~~

(306)

If we don't want to work it off, let's not eat it.

~~~~~~~~~~

(307)

Make a total commitment to losing weight or don't bother trying. There is no half way.

~~~~~~~~~~

(308)

Weight-loss excuses will rob us of a healthy future if we let them.

(309)

We can feel our best just by losing some weight. If we look our best,
we will feel our best.

~~~~~~~~~~

(310)

We should prefer weight-loss failure over not starting at all.

~~~~~~~~~~

(311)

If we keep eating what we want, when we want, we will end up where
we don't want.

~~~~~~~~~~

(312)

We are overweight because of the things we did and did not do to get
there.

(313)

What price will we pay for being overweight? Will we pay with our lives maybe? Losing weight may be easier.

~~~~~~~~~

(314)

Let's not accept being overweight, unless we want an unhealthy future.

~~~~~~~~~

(315)

Let's use exercise as time for ourselves.

~~~~~~~~~

(316)

Say "Yes" to a healthier future and "No" to anything that will keep us from the future we want.

(317)

Getting thinner will make us happier. If we enjoy the process, we will stay thinner.

~~~~~~~~~~

(318)

Let's not look for the magic pill to help us lose weight. There isn't one.

~~~~~~~~~~

(319)

The more overweight we are, the more we will eventually be hurt by our weight.

~~~~~~~~~~

(320)

Getting and staying thin is all about balancing the foods we love with healthy foods.

(321)

If exercise reduces heart disease, stroke, diabetes, obesity, and osteoporosis why would we want to avoid exercise?

~~~~~~~~~~

(322)

To change our weight, we must change some of our habits.

~~~~~~~~~~

(323)

Our health is the most important thing we have. What are we doing to take care of it?

~~~~~~~~~~

(324)

If we don't watch what we eat and how much we eat, the only things we will be watching is our weight go up and our health go down.

(325)

Don't have any regrets. There are people in the hospital wishing they lost weight and took better care of their health.

~~~~~~~~~

(326)

What went in our mouths caused our weight today. What we decide to put in our mouths from this point on will decide our weight in the future.

~~~~~~~~~

(327)

Do your knees hurt? Does it take effort to get out of the chair? Do you think moving around would be easier if you were thinner? Your body is telling you to lose weight. The issue is whether you hear it.

~~~~~~~~~

(328)

Weight loss is the result of not eating everything and anything we want, when we want it.

(329)

Every day, we should ask ourselves this question, "How am I going to show my commitment to losing weight today?"

~~~~~~~~~~

(330)

We should ask ourselves in every situation, "Would a thin person do this?"

~~~~~~~~~~

(331)

The thin person thinks of reasons to stay thin. An overweight person thinks of excuses to stay overweight. Which are you?

~~~~~~~~~~

(332)

We need to ask ourselves whether we just want to live or whether we want to live a longer and healthier life?

(333)

Give 100 percent of your attention and priority to losing weight. I did this when I was in the weight-loss process for 4 months and it worked.

~~~~~~~~~~

(334)

Always say "No" to overeating.

~~~~~~~~~~

(335)

If we can let go of our bad habits, we will let go of our weight.

~~~~~~~~~~

(336)

The road of "Staying Overweight" is also called "The Road to Bad Health." Stay off this road.

(337)

We fail at losing weight when we place a higher importance on other things.

~~~~~~~~~~

(338)

If we can develop restraint, we can become thinner. Restraint is a habit that can be developed.

~~~~~~~~~~

(339)

I would rather have a little weight-loss success than no success at all.

~~~~~~~~~~

(340)

A habit is something we do over and over. It becomes part of us. Let's make regular exercise a habit. Let's make eating less and eating healthier a habit. These changes will become easier as they become part of us.

(341)

Everyday, let's modify our bad habits slowly and watch the weight come off.

~~~~~~~~~~

(342)

We gained our weight when we gained our bad habits. We will lose our weight when we lose our bad habits.

~~~~~~~~~~

(343)

Our brain tells our body what to do. Our brain tells our body to go into the fast-food restaurant and triple-size. Let's start telling our body to exercise and eat healthier.

~~~~~~~~~~

(344)

If we can develop a thin person mind-set, we will be able to lose weight and keep it off for a lifetime.

(345)

Learn why and how we gained the weight and then do the opposite.

~~~~~~~~~~~

(346)

An overweight person looks for every excuse not to exercise. A thin person looks for every opportunity to get exercise throughout the day.

~~~~~~~~~~~

(347)

It really is easier to be thinner than overweight. Try it, you will like it.

~~~~~~~~~~~

(348)

Health problems that will happen because of our weight may not be able to be reversed. Reduce the risk of having these problems by starting to lose weight today.

(349)

Developing a thin mindset will allow us to consistently make thin choices. Making thin choices consistently will allow us to become thinner.

~~~~~~~~~~

(350)

If we don't like our weight, we can change it, or we can end up where we don't want to be.

~~~~~~~~~~

(351)

Boredom and stress are two enemies of weight loss because they drive most people to eat.

~~~~~~~~~~

(352)

How thin people and overweight people think about food, and exercise are totally opposite. Hence, their results are totally opposite. If we change how we think about food and exercise, our results will change.

(353)

A weight-loss goal consists of the weight we want to be, and the date we want to reach that weight. Let's set a realistic goal and let's start today.

~~~~~~~~~~

(354)

Having a sense of urgency towards weight loss will allow you to win at weight loss.

~~~~~~~~~~

(355)

Most reasons people give for not losing weight are nothing but excuses for not doing what they know they should be doing.

~~~~~~~~~~

(356)

Being overweight is not the problem. The problem is not doing anything about it.

(357)

Once we hit our weight-loss goal it is always a good idea to set another goal. Set a goal of getting fitter. Set a goal of losing more weight. This can keep the motivation going.

~~~~~~~~~~

(358)

We became overweight not by overeating once but by doing it many times. We lose weight by under eating many times.

~~~~~~~~~~

(359)

If we want to become thinner, we will need to have total commitment to our weight loss, health, and fitness. If we are unwilling to give our full commitment, we should look forward to an unhealthy future.

~~~~~~~~~~

(360)

An obstacle is a bump in the road we can get around. A weight-loss obstacle is a bump in the road to losing weight that we can also get around. Remember, it would not be called an obstacle if we could not get around it.

(361)

It is okay to lose weight slowly as long as we don't stop until we reach our goal.

~~~~~~~~~

(362)

Get rid of our denial and start living our dream of being thinner.

~~~~~~~~~

(363)

We can have the weight we want to have. We just have to do the work.

~~~~~~~~~

(364)

Are we at the weight we want? It is doable if we truly want it.

(365)

If we think we can't lose weight, we may need to increase our effort.

Extra Nibbles

Extra Nibbles

A Friend of mine named Eric, who is a firefighter told me this one. "We need to get thinner before we get older because someone will have to move us around." His daily experience as a firefighter, has taught him that one. "The thinner we are the less our families will have to call 911."

~~~~~~~~~~~

We should weigh ourselves daily to help us stay focused.

~~~~~~~~~~~

Put a plan together for the obstacles we will encounter.

~~~~~~~~~~~

At the end of each day of losing weight we need to ask ourselves, "Do I feel good about the choices I made today? Do I feel that I deprived myself of anything?" If we don't feel good about the choices we've made, and we feel that we've deprived ourselves, then we need to change what we are doing. We won't lose weight for a lifetime going through each day thinking that we have deprived ourselves.

Rules to Live by

When I was in the weight loss process, I found myself making a few general rules I committed to live by. These rules helped guide my decisions and gave me strength to overcome temptation when I walked into various situations.

Here are a few rules I made:

- I pack my lunch. If a lunch is brought from home, people will have more control over what they eat, and the temptation for eating junk is removed.

- I don't eat French fries at lunchtime. This one is for the rare occasions I do eat out for lunch. When in this situation, I substitute a side of fruit for anything that comes with fries. I am not saying that I gave up French fries totally. I just committed not to eat them at lunch. If I am out for dinner, and ate a healthy and light breakfast and lunch, I can eat the fries, I just watch the quantity I eat.

- I limit alcoholic drinks to two on the weekends. Alcoholic drinks are full of calories that can add on pounds.

- I like to get calories from foods I eat, not drink. It is always a good idea to reduce or eliminate sugary sodas and juices from our daily routine. There are many low/no calorie drinks on the market that can be substituted.

- I exercise daily. Even taking a 20 to 30 minute walk at lunch would be a benefit.

- I stopped the seconds. This one should be quite obvious. Make it a rule not to go up for second plates of food.

These are some of the general rules I live by.

Sometimes I break the rules but when I do, I am careful and aware of it. I make sure I have been cautious with my other meals before breaking one of the rules.

Check out my "Two-Thirds Rule" on the next page. It has worked extremely well for me over the years. It is definitely something to consider.

If we want to lose weight, we need to make some general rules for ourselves.

My "Two-Thirds Eating Rule"

When I first started the weight-loss processes, I did what a lot of people do. I starved my and gave up all my favorite foods. This did nothing but frustrate me. One day I thought to myself, "This will not work. I can't do this long term. I need to create a way that I can have a balanced approach to losing weight so that I can lose it and keep it off. I needed to create an approach that I could eat healthier and still enjoy my favorite foods."

Hence, through trial and error, I created what I like to call my "Two-Thirds Rule"

 What I did and still do is this. I make sure that at least two-thirds of my meals and snacks are healthy. The other third of my meals and snack may be healthy, or may be my favorite comfort foods (in smaller portions).

This allows me to eat healthier, eat my favorite foods in limited quantities, and it allows me not to feel deprived. It is a long-term strategy that I used to drop 50 pounds in four months and keep it off for over seven years.

This may not work for everyone; however, it has worked for me and many other people I have helped.

Goal Sheet for Losing Weight

My current weight: _____

My goal weight: _____

When am I going to start (now is a good time)? _____

What date will I lose the weight by? _____

What is my core reason for losing weight (My Reason Why)?

_____

_____

What am I willing to do to get to this weight? (This shows my commitment level.)

_____

_____

Is there a specific area I want to concentrate on? _____

What am I going to do in the next 12 hours towards the above weight-loss goal? (This shows I'm serious.)

Page Reprinted from *Don't Diet! Just Think And Get Thin* by George A. Diamond

The Day After
Daily Weight-Loss Journal
(Everyday I weigh myself and then ask myself the questions below)

What was my weight yesterday: _____
What is my weight today: _____

Was my weight Lower / Same / Higher than yesterday?

Am I happy with the direction that my weight went?

Did I exercise yesterday?

Was my activity level Low / Medium / High yesterday?

What type of foods did I eat yesterday?

How were my portion sizes yesterday?

What did I do correctly yesterday that I can repeat today?

What can I do differently today to achieve my weight-loss goal?

Did I feel that I deprived myself of anything yesterday?

This Weight-Loss Action Form will assist us with our
weight-loss plan.

Weight-Loss Action Form

What **actions** we are going to take: Goal Date:

1. _____   1. _____

   _____

2. _____   2. _____

   _____

3. _____   3. _____

   _____

4. _____   4. _____

Results:

Short-Term Goals (1 week):

Long-Term Goals:

What obstacles are anticipated?

How are we going to overcome the above obstacles?

Cost: (What are we willing to give, such as time, money, and commitment?)

Page Reprinted from *Don't Diet! Just Think And Get Thin* by George A. Diamond

Which one of these actions can we take today to move towards our goal of losing weight and getting fitter? If the hardest thing to do is to start, which of these actions can we start today? Let's start the process by showing our commitment and take the first steps towards a thinner and healthier future.

Page Reprinted from *Don't Diet! Just Think And Get Thin* by George A. Diamond

The list below illustrates two points:

1) What **excuses** for not losing weight can result in.
2) What **reasons** for losing weight can result in (if followed by actions).

Excuses Can Result In

Overweight, Obesity
Poor Health, Sickness
High Blood Pressure
High Cholesterol, Cancer
Diabetes, Heart Attack
Pills, Shots, Stroke, Death
Immobility, Hospitals
Pain, Sorrow, Loss, Grief
Financial Ruin
Lost Relationships

Reasons Can Result In

Being Thinner, Fitter, Longer Life
Good Health, Mobility
Lower Blood Pressure, Good Appearance
Higher Energy
Success
Self-Confidence

About the Author

As a graduate of Wayne State University with my B.S. in Electrical Engineering, I was trained in solving problems. In my first job after college, I developed engineering and manufacturing software for a large automotive manufacturer. In my next position I worked in the same capacity as well as in business systems development for a big automotive supplier. Along the way, I started a computer company that designs systems, fixes IT problems, teaches computer skills, and develops software and websites.

What does that have to do with losing weight?

Two important things:
1) I applied the same objective problem-solving skills I learned in college to solve my weight problem, lose 50 pounds in 4 months, and have kept it off for seven years.

2) I used my experience of analyzing and developing systems to develop a system that anyone who desires to lose weight can use.

Now, add to that the passion I have to teach, and my weight-loss system was born.

Visit

NibblesOfEncouragement.com

Check out George's Other Book
Don't Diet! Just Think And Get Thin
At
DontDietJustThink.com

More Weight-Loss Resources
Visit
LoseWeightFastWithoutDieting.com

www.ingramcontent.com/pod-product-compliance
Lightning Source LLC
Chambersburg PA
CBHW072007060426
42446CB00042B/2019